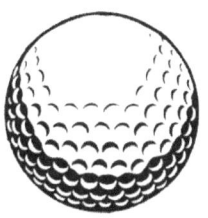

IF FOUND PLEASE CONTACT

_____

_____

_____

DEDICATION

This book is dedicated to all the Golfers out there.

You are my inspiration in producing books for golfers, especially to record "braggin' rights" memories that will last a lifetime.

How To Use This Pocket Golf Score Log Book:

This ultimate pocket golf score notebook is a perfect way to track and record all your favorite golf games. This unique golf score notebook is a great way to keep your golfing information all in one place.

Each interior page includes prompts and space to record the following:

1. Course - Write the name of the golf course.

2. Location - Write out where you played.

3. Date - What day you played.

4. Weather - Record what the weather was that day.

5. Players - Stay on task by naming all the players in your group... come back here later to have a good laugh...

6. Par - Record the number of strokes per hole.

7. Stroke - Keep track of how many times to hit the ball.

8. Fairway - Track any hazards along the way.

9. Putts - Write in how many strokes were made.

10. Hazards - Track any trees, obstacles, bunkers along the way.

11. Score - Keep score for every round of golf.

If you are new to the game of golf, or have been at this for a while...this golf pocket planner is a must have! Can make an awesome gift for the golf lover, and will be a keepsake forever.

Enjoy!

COURSE		LOCATION	
DATE		WEATHER	
PLAYERS			

	1	2	3	4	5	6	7	8	9	TOTAL
PAR										
STROKE										
FAIRWAY										
PUTTS										
HAZARDS										
+/-										
SCORE										

	10	11	12	13	14	15	16	17	18	TOTAL
PAR										
STROKE										
FAIRWAY										
PUTTS										
HAZARDS										
+/-										
SCORE										

NOTES

COURSE		LOCATION	
DATE		WEATHER	
PLAYERS			

	1	2	3	4	5	6	7	8	9	TOTAL
PAR										
STROKE										
FAIRWAY										
PUTTS										
HAZARDS										
+/-										
SCORE										

	10	11	12	13	14	15	16	17	18	TOTAL
PAR										
STROKE										
FAIRWAY										
PUTTS										
HAZARDS										
+/-										
SCORE										

NOTES

COURSE	LOCATION
DATE	WEATHER

PLAYERS

	1	2	3	4	5	6	7	8	9	TOTAL
PAR										
STROKE										
FAIRWAY										
PUTTS										
HAZARDS										
+/-										
SCORE										

	10	11	12	13	14	15	16	17	18	TOTAL
PAR										
STROKE										
FAIRWAY										
PUTTS										
HAZARDS										
+/-										
SCORE										

NOTES

COURSE		LOCATION	
DATE		WEATHER	
PLAYERS			

	1	2	3	4	5	6	7	8	9	TOTAL
PAR										
STROKE										
FAIRWAY										
PUTTS										
HAZARDS										
+/-										
SCORE										

	10	11	12	13	14	15	16	17	18	TOTAL
PAR										
STROKE										
FAIRWAY										
PUTTS										
HAZARDS										
+/-										
SCORE										

NOTES

COURSE

LOCATION

DATE

WEATHER

PLAYERS

	1	2	3	4	5	6	7	8	9	TOTAL
PAR										
STROKE										
FAIRWAY										
PUTTS										
HAZARDS										
+/-										
SCORE										

	10	11	12	13	14	15	16	17	18	TOTAL
PAR										
STROKE										
FAIRWAY										
PUTTS										
HAZARDS										
+/-										
SCORE										

NOTES

COURSE		LOCATION	
DATE		WEATHER	
PLAYERS			

	1	2	3	4	5	6	7	8	9	TOTAL
PAR										
STROKE										
FAIRWAY										
PUTTS										
HAZARDS										
+/-										
SCORE										

	10	11	12	13	14	15	16	17	18	TOTAL
PAR										
STROKE										
FAIRWAY										
PUTTS										
HAZARDS										
+/-										
SCORE										

NOTES

COURSE	LOCATION
DATE	WEATHER

PLAYERS

	1	2	3	4	5	6	7	8	9	TOTAL
PAR										
STROKE										
FAIRWAY										
PUTTS										
HAZARDS										
+/-										
SCORE										

	10	11	12	13	14	15	16	17	18	TOTAL
PAR										
STROKE										
FAIRWAY										
PUTTS										
HAZARDS										
+/-										
SCORE										

NOTES

COURSE		LOCATION	
DATE		WEATHER	

PLAYERS

	1	2	3	4	5	6	7	8	9	TOTAL
PAR										
STROKE										
FAIRWAY										
PUTTS										
HAZARDS										
+/-										
SCORE										

	10	11	12	13	14	15	16	17	18	TOTAL
PAR										
STROKE										
FAIRWAY										
PUTTS										
HAZARDS										
+/-										
SCORE										

NOTES

COURSE

LOCATION

DATE

WEATHER

PLAYERS

	1	2	3	4	5	6	7	8	9	TOTAL
PAR										
STROKE										
FAIRWAY										
PUTTS										
HAZARDS										
+/-										
SCORE										

	10	11	12	13	14	15	16	17	18	TOTAL
PAR										
STROKE										
FAIRWAY										
PUTTS										
HAZARDS										
+/-										
SCORE										

NOTES

COURSE

LOCATION

DATE

WEATHER

PLAYERS

	1	2	3	4	5	6	7	8	9	TOTAL
PAR										
STROKE										
FAIRWAY										
PUTTS										
HAZARDS										
+/-										
SCORE										

	10	11	12	13	14	15	16	17	18	TOTAL
PAR										
STROKE										
FAIRWAY										
PUTTS										
HAZARDS										
+/-										
SCORE										

NOTES

COURSE		LOCATION	
DATE		WEATHER	
PLAYERS			

	1	2	3	4	5	6	7	8	9	TOTAL
PAR										
STROKE										
FAIRWAY										
PUTTS										
HAZARDS										
+/-										
SCORE										

	10	11	12	13	14	15	16	17	18	TOTAL
PAR										
STROKE										
FAIRWAY										
PUTTS										
HAZARDS										
+/-										
SCORE										

NOTES

COURSE

LOCATION

DATE

WEATHER

PLAYERS

	1	2	3	4	5	6	7	8	9	TOTAL
PAR										
STROKE										
FAIRWAY										
PUTTS										
HAZARDS										
+/-										
SCORE										

	10	11	12	13	14	15	16	17	18	TOTAL
PAR										
STROKE										
FAIRWAY										
PUTTS										
HAZARDS										
+/-										
SCORE										

NOTES

COURSE		LOCATION	
DATE		WEATHER	
PLAYERS			

	1	2	3	4	5	6	7	8	9	TOTAL
PAR										
STROKE										
FAIRWAY										
PUTTS										
HAZARDS										
+/-										
SCORE										

	10	11	12	13	14	15	16	17	18	TOTAL
PAR										
STROKE										
FAIRWAY										
PUTTS										
HAZARDS										
+/-										
SCORE										

NOTES

COURSE

LOCATION

DATE

WEATHER

PLAYERS

	1	2	3	4	5	6	7	8	9	TOTAL
PAR										
STROKE										
FAIRWAY										
PUTTS										
HAZARDS										
+/-										
SCORE										

	10	11	12	13	14	15	16	17	18	TOTAL
PAR										
STROKE										
FAIRWAY										
PUTTS										
HAZARDS										
+/-										
SCORE										

NOTES

COURSE

LOCATION

DATE

WEATHER

PLAYERS

	1	2	3	4	5	6	7	8	9	TOTAL
PAR										
STROKE										
FAIRWAY										
PUTTS										
HAZARDS										
+/-										
SCORE										

	10	11	12	13	14	15	16	17	18	TOTAL
PAR										
STROKE										
FAIRWAY										
PUTTS										
HAZARDS										
+/-										
SCORE										

NOTES

COURSE		LOCATION	
DATE		WEATHER	
PLAYERS			

	1	2	3	4	5	6	7	8	9	TOTAL
PAR										
STROKE										
FAIRWAY										
PUTTS										
HAZARDS										
+/-										
SCORE										

	10	11	12	13	14	15	16	17	18	TOTAL
PAR										
STROKE										
FAIRWAY										
PUTTS										
HAZARDS										
+/-										
SCORE										

NOTES

COURSE									LOCATION	
DATE									WEATHER	
PLAYERS										

	1	2	3	4	5	6	7	8	9	TOTAL
PAR										
STROKE										
FAIRWAY										
PUTTS										
HAZARDS										
+/-										
SCORE										

	10	11	12	13	14	15	16	17	18	TOTAL
PAR										
STROKE										
FAIRWAY										
PUTTS										
HAZARDS										
+/-										
SCORE										

NOTES

COURSE		LOCATION	
DATE		WEATHER	
PLAYERS			

	1	2	3	4	5	6	7	8	9	TOTAL
PAR										
STROKE										
FAIRWAY										
PUTTS										
HAZARDS										
+/-										
SCORE										

	10	11	12	13	14	15	16	17	18	TOTAL
PAR										
STROKE										
FAIRWAY										
PUTTS										
HAZARDS										
+/-										
SCORE										

NOTES

COURSE		LOCATION	
DATE		WEATHER	
PLAYERS			

	1	2	3	4	5	6	7	8	9	TOTAL
PAR										
STROKE										
FAIRWAY										
PUTTS										
HAZARDS										
+/-										
SCORE										

	10	11	12	13	14	15	16	17	18	TOTAL
PAR										
STROKE										
FAIRWAY										
PUTTS										
HAZARDS										
+/-										
SCORE										

NOTES

COURSE		LOCATION	
DATE		WEATHER	
PLAYERS			

	1	2	3	4	5	6	7	8	9	TOTAL
PAR										
STROKE										
FAIRWAY										
PUTTS										
HAZARDS										
+/-										
SCORE										

	10	11	12	13	14	15	16	17	18	TOTAL
PAR										
STROKE										
FAIRWAY										
PUTTS										
HAZARDS										
+/-										
SCORE										

NOTES

COURSE
DATE
PLAYERS

LOCATION
WEATHER

	1	2	3	4	5	6	7	8	9	TOTAL
PAR										
STROKE										
FAIRWAY										
PUTTS										
HAZARDS										
+/-										
SCORE										

	10	11	12	13	14	15	16	17	18	TOTAL
PAR										
STROKE										
FAIRWAY										
PUTTS										
HAZARDS										
+/-										
SCORE										

NOTES

COURSE

LOCATION

DATE

WEATHER

PLAYERS

	1	2	3	4	5	6	7	8	9	TOTAL
PAR										
STROKE										
FAIRWAY										
PUTTS										
HAZARDS										
+/-										
SCORE										

	10	11	12	13	14	15	16	17	18	TOTAL
PAR										
STROKE										
FAIRWAY										
PUTTS										
HAZARDS										
+/-										
SCORE										

NOTES

COURSE										LOCATION
DATE										WEATHER

PLAYERS

	1	2	3	4	5	6	7	8	9	TOTAL
PAR										
STROKE										
FAIRWAY										
PUTTS										
HAZARDS										
+/-										
SCORE										

	10	11	12	13	14	15	16	17	18	TOTAL
PAR										
STROKE										
FAIRWAY										
PUTTS										
HAZARDS										
+/-										
SCORE										

NOTES

COURSE

LOCATION

DATE

WEATHER

PLAYERS

	1	2	3	4	5	6	7	8	9	TOTAL
PAR										
STROKE										
FAIRWAY										
PUTTS										
HAZARDS										
+/-										
SCORE										

	10	11	12	13	14	15	16	17	18	TOTAL
PAR										
STROKE										
FAIRWAY										
PUTTS										
HAZARDS										
+/-										
SCORE										

NOTES

COURSE	LOCATION
DATE	WEATHER
PLAYERS	

	1	2	3	4	5	6	7	8	9	TOTAL
PAR										
STROKE										
FAIRWAY										
PUTTS										
HAZARDS										
+/-										
SCORE										

	10	11	12	13	14	15	16	17	18	TOTAL
PAR										
STROKE										
FAIRWAY										
PUTTS										
HAZARDS										
+/-										
SCORE										

NOTES

COURSE		LOCATION	
DATE		WEATHER	
PLAYERS			

	1	2	3	4	5	6	7	8	9	TOTAL
PAR										
STROKE										
FAIRWAY										
PUTTS										
HAZARDS										
+/-										
SCORE										

	10	11	12	13	14	15	16	17	18	TOTAL
PAR										
STROKE										
FAIRWAY										
PUTTS										
HAZARDS										
+/-										
SCORE										

NOTES

COURSE	LOCATION
DATE	WEATHER
PLAYERS	

	1	2	3	4	5	6	7	8	9	TOTAL
PAR										
STROKE										
FAIRWAY										
PUTTS										
HAZARDS										
+/-										
SCORE										

	10	11	12	13	14	15	16	17	18	TOTAL
PAR										
STROKE										
FAIRWAY										
PUTTS										
HAZARDS										
+/-										
SCORE										

NOTES

COURSE

LOCATION

DATE

WEATHER

PLAYERS

	1	2	3	4	5	6	7	8	9	TOTAL
PAR										
STROKE										
FAIRWAY										
PUTTS										
HAZARDS										
+/-										
SCORE										

	10	11	12	13	14	15	16	17	18	TOTAL
PAR										
STROKE										
FAIRWAY										
PUTTS										
HAZARDS										
+/-										
SCORE										

NOTES

COURSE

LOCATION

DATE

WEATHER

PLAYERS

	1	2	3	4	5	6	7	8	9	TOTAL
PAR										
STROKE										
FAIRWAY										
PUTTS										
HAZARDS										
+/-										
SCORE										

	10	11	12	13	14	15	16	17	18	TOTAL
PAR										
STROKE										
FAIRWAY										
PUTTS										
HAZARDS										
+/-										
SCORE										

NOTES

COURSE

LOCATION

DATE

WEATHER

PLAYERS

	1	2	3	4	5	6	7	8	9	TOTAL
PAR										
STROKE										
FAIRWAY										
PUTTS										
HAZARDS										
+/-										
SCORE										

	10	11	12	13	14	15	16	17	18	TOTAL
PAR										
STROKE										
FAIRWAY										
PUTTS										
HAZARDS										
+/-										
SCORE										

NOTES

COURSE		LOCATION	
DATE		WEATHER	
PLAYERS			

	1	2	3	4	5	6	7	8	9	TOTAL
PAR										
STROKE										
FAIRWAY										
PUTTS										
HAZARDS										
+/-										
SCORE										

	10	11	12	13	14	15	16	17	18	TOTAL
PAR										
STROKE										
FAIRWAY										
PUTTS										
HAZARDS										
+/-										
SCORE										

NOTES

COURSE		LOCATION	
DATE		WEATHER	
PLAYERS			

	1	2	3	4	5	6	7	8	9	TOTAL
PAR										
STROKE										
FAIRWAY										
PUTTS										
HAZARDS										
+/-										
SCORE										

	10	11	12	13	14	15	16	17	18	TOTAL
PAR										
STROKE										
FAIRWAY										
PUTTS										
HAZARDS										
+/-										
SCORE										

NOTES

COURSE	LOCATION
DATE	WEATHER
PLAYERS	

	1	2	3	4	5	6	7	8	9	TOTAL
PAR										
STROKE										
FAIRWAY										
PUTTS										
HAZARDS										
+/-										
SCORE										

	10	11	12	13	14	15	16	17	18	TOTAL
PAR										
STROKE										
FAIRWAY										
PUTTS										
HAZARDS										
+/-										
SCORE										

NOTES

COURSE

LOCATION

DATE

WEATHER

PLAYERS

	1	2	3	4	5	6	7	8	9	TOTAL
PAR										
STROKE										
FAIRWAY										
PUTTS										
HAZARDS										
+/-										
SCORE										

	10	11	12	13	14	15	16	17	18	TOTAL
PAR										
STROKE										
FAIRWAY										
PUTTS										
HAZARDS										
+/-										
SCORE										

NOTES

COURSE		LOCATION	
DATE		WEATHER	
PLAYERS			

	1	2	3	4	5	6	7	8	9	TOTAL
PAR										
STROKE										
FAIRWAY										
PUTTS										
HAZARDS										
+/-										
SCORE										

	10	11	12	13	14	15	16	17	18	TOTAL
PAR										
STROKE										
FAIRWAY										
PUTTS										
HAZARDS										
+/-										
SCORE										

NOTES

COURSE		LOCATION	
DATE		WEATHER	
PLAYERS			

	1	2	3	4	5	6	7	8	9	TOTAL
PAR										
STROKE										
FAIRWAY										
PUTTS										
HAZARDS										
+/-										
SCORE										

	10	11	12	13	14	15	16	17	18	TOTAL
PAR										
STROKE										
FAIRWAY										
PUTTS										
HAZARDS										
+/-										
SCORE										

NOTES

COURSE	LOCATION
DATE	WEATHER

PLAYERS

	1	2	3	4	5	6	7	8	9	TOTAL
PAR										
STROKE										
FAIRWAY										
PUTTS										
HAZARDS										
+/-										
SCORE										

	10	11	12	13	14	15	16	17	18	TOTAL
PAR										
STROKE										
FAIRWAY										
PUTTS										
HAZARDS										
+/-										
SCORE										

NOTES

COURSE	LOCATION
DATE	WEATHER
PLAYERS	

	1	2	3	4	5	6	7	8	9	TOTAL
PAR										
STROKE										
FAIRWAY										
PUTTS										
HAZARDS										
+/-										
SCORE										

	10	11	12	13	14	15	16	17	18	TOTAL
PAR										
STROKE										
FAIRWAY										
PUTTS										
HAZARDS										
+/-										
SCORE										

NOTES

COURSE

LOCATION

DATE

WEATHER

PLAYERS

	1	2	3	4	5	6	7	8	9	TOTAL
PAR										
STROKE										
FAIRWAY										
PUTTS										
HAZARDS										
+/-										
SCORE										

	10	11	12	13	14	15	16	17	18	TOTAL
PAR										
STROKE										
FAIRWAY										
PUTTS										
HAZARDS										
+/-										
SCORE										

NOTES

COURSE		LOCATION	
DATE		WEATHER	|️
PLAYERS			

	1	2	3	4	5	6	7	8	9	TOTAL
PAR										
STROKE										
FAIRWAY										
PUTTS										
HAZARDS										
+/-										
SCORE										

	10	11	12	13	14	15	16	17	18	TOTAL
PAR										
STROKE										
FAIRWAY										
PUTTS										
HAZARDS										
+/-										
SCORE										

NOTES

COURSE

LOCATION

DATE

WEATHER

PLAYERS

	1	2	3	4	5	6	7	8	9	TOTAL
PAR										
STROKE										
FAIRWAY										
PUTTS										
HAZARDS										
+/-										
SCORE										

	10	11	12	13	14	15	16	17	18	TOTAL
PAR										
STROKE										
FAIRWAY										
PUTTS										
HAZARDS										
+/-										
SCORE										

NOTES

COURSE									
DATE									
PLAYERS									

LOCATION	
WEATHER	

	1	2	3	4	5	6	7	8	9	TOTAL
PAR										
STROKE										
FAIRWAY										
PUTTS										
HAZARDS										
+/-										
SCORE										

	10	11	12	13	14	15	16	17	18	TOTAL
PAR										
STROKE										
FAIRWAY										
PUTTS										
HAZARDS										
+/-										
SCORE										

NOTES

COURSE		LOCATION	
DATE		WEATHER	
PLAYERS			

	1	2	3	4	5	6	7	8	9	TOTAL
PAR										
STROKE										
FAIRWAY										
PUTTS										
HAZARDS										
+/-										
SCORE										

	10	11	12	13	14	15	16	17	18	TOTAL
PAR										
STROKE										
FAIRWAY										
PUTTS										
HAZARDS										
+/-										
SCORE										

NOTES

COURSE		LOCATION	
DATE		WEATHER	
PLAYERS			

	1	2	3	4	5	6	7	8	9	TOTAL
PAR										
STROKE										
FAIRWAY										
PUTTS										
HAZARDS										
+/-										
SCORE										

	10	11	12	13	14	15	16	17	18	TOTAL
PAR										
STROKE										
FAIRWAY										
PUTTS										
HAZARDS										
+/-										
SCORE										

NOTES

COURSE		LOCATION	
DATE		WEATHER	
PLAYERS			

	1	2	3	4	5	6	7	8	9	TOTAL
PAR										
STROKE										
FAIRWAY										
PUTTS										
HAZARDS										
+/-										
SCORE										

	10	11	12	13	14	15	16	17	18	TOTAL
PAR										
STROKE										
FAIRWAY										
PUTTS										
HAZARDS										
+/-										
SCORE										

NOTES

COURSE		LOCATION	
DATE		WEATHER	
PLAYERS			

	1	2	3	4	5	6	7	8	9	TOTAL
PAR										
STROKE										
FAIRWAY										
PUTTS										
HAZARDS										
+/-										
SCORE										

	10	11	12	13	14	15	16	17	18	TOTAL
PAR										
STROKE										
FAIRWAY										
PUTTS										
HAZARDS										
+/-										
SCORE										

NOTES

COURSE

LOCATION

DATE

WEATHER

PLAYERS

	1	2	3	4	5	6	7	8	9	TOTAL
PAR										
STROKE										
FAIRWAY										
PUTTS										
HAZARDS										
+/-										
SCORE										

	10	11	12	13	14	15	16	17	18	TOTAL
PAR										
STROKE										
FAIRWAY										
PUTTS										
HAZARDS										
+/-										
SCORE										

NOTES

COURSE

LOCATION

DATE

WEATHER

PLAYERS

	1	2	3	4	5	6	7	8	9	TOTAL
PAR										
STROKE										
FAIRWAY										
PUTTS										
HAZARDS										
+/-										
SCORE										

	10	11	12	13	14	15	16	17	18	TOTAL
PAR										
STROKE										
FAIRWAY										
PUTTS										
HAZARDS										
+/-										
SCORE										

NOTES

COURSE

LOCATION

DATE

WEATHER

PLAYERS

	1	2	3	4	5	6	7	8	9	TOTAL
PAR										
STROKE										
FAIRWAY										
PUTTS										
HAZARDS										
+/-										
SCORE										

	10	11	12	13	14	15	16	17	18	TOTAL
PAR										
STROKE										
FAIRWAY										
PUTTS										
HAZARDS										
+/-										
SCORE										

NOTES

COURSE

LOCATION

DATE

WEATHER

PLAYERS

	1	2	3	4	5	6	7	8	9	TOTAL
PAR										
STROKE										
FAIRWAY										
PUTTS										
HAZARDS										
+/-										
SCORE										

	10	11	12	13	14	15	16	17	18	TOTAL
PAR										
STROKE										
FAIRWAY										
PUTTS										
HAZARDS										
+/-										
SCORE										

NOTES

COURSE		LOCATION	
DATE		WEATHER	
PLAYERS			

	1	2	3	4	5	6	7	8	9	TOTAL
PAR										
STROKE										
FAIRWAY										
PUTTS										
HAZARDS										
+/-										
SCORE										

	10	11	12	13	14	15	16	17	18	TOTAL
PAR										
STROKE										
FAIRWAY										
PUTTS										
HAZARDS										
+/-										
SCORE										

NOTES

COURSE		LOCATION	
DATE		WEATHER	
PLAYERS			

	1	2	3	4	5	6	7	8	9	TOTAL
PAR										
STROKE										
FAIRWAY										
PUTTS										
HAZARDS										
+/-										
SCORE										

	10	11	12	13	14	15	16	17	18	TOTAL
PAR										
STROKE										
FAIRWAY										
PUTTS										
HAZARDS										
+/-										
SCORE										

NOTES

COURSE		LOCATION	
DATE		WEATHER	
PLAYERS			

	1	2	3	4	5	6	7	8	9	TOTAL
PAR										
STROKE										
FAIRWAY										
PUTTS										
HAZARDS										
+/-										
SCORE										

	10	11	12	13	14	15	16	17	18	TOTAL
PAR										
STROKE										
FAIRWAY										
PUTTS										
HAZARDS										
+/-										
SCORE										

NOTES

COURSE

LOCATION

DATE

WEATHER

PLAYERS

	1	2	3	4	5	6	7	8	9	TOTAL
PAR										
STROKE										
FAIRWAY										
PUTTS										
HAZARDS										
+/-										
SCORE										

	10	11	12	13	14	15	16	17	18	TOTAL
PAR										
STROKE										
FAIRWAY										
PUTTS										
HAZARDS										
+/-										
SCORE										

www.ingramcontent.com/pod-product-compliance
Lightning Source LLC
Chambersburg PA
CBHW071250070526
44583CB00017B/2402